Table of Contents

Each chapter will dive into the topic, providing practical exercises, tips, case studies, and insights from experts in the field. By the end, readers would have a comprehensive guide to Pilates, suitable for beginners and seasoned practitioners alike.

Chapter 1: Introduction

Pilates: A Journey to Mindful Movement

In the bustling world we inhabit, finding moments of tranquility and connection can seem like an elusive dream. Yet, nestled within the realm of mindful movement lies a practice that offers not only physical strength and flexibility but also a pathway to inner harmony and balance. Welcome to the world of Pilates.

In this introductory chapter, we embark on a journey to explore the origins, principles, and transformative power of Pilates. From its humble beginnings in the early 20th century to its widespread popularity in the modern age, Pilates has evolved into a holistic approach to fitness and wellbeing.

Origins of Pilates

Our journey begins with a glimpse into the life of Joseph Pilates, the visionary creator of this method. Born in Germany in 1883, Pilates overcome personal adversity and dedicated his life to understanding the intricate connection between mind, body, and spirit. Influenced by various disciplines such as yoga, gymnastics, and martial arts, he developed a series of exercises designed to enhance physical strength, flexibility, and alignment.

Principles of Pilates

Central to the Pilates method are its guiding principles, which form the foundation of every movement and breath. From the concept of centering, where attention is drawn to the core muscles, to the emphasis on precision and control, each principle serves to unite mind and body in harmonious synergy. Throughout this book, we will explore these principles in depth, unlocking the secrets to mastering the art of Pilates.

The Transformative Power of Pilates

Beyond its physical benefits, Pilates offers a pathway to transformation on a deeper level. Through mindful movement and breath awareness, practitioners cultivate a sense of presence and mindfulness that extends beyond the mat and into everyday life. Whether you are seeking to alleviate back pain, enhance athletic performance, or simply reconnect with your body, Pilates offers a sanctuary where mind, body, and spirit converge in perfect harmony.

As we embark on this journey together, may you discover the joy of Pilates and the infinite possibilities that await within. Let us begin, with open hearts and open minds, on the path to mindful movement and inner transformation.

Chapter 2: Understanding the Core

In the vast landscape of fitness, the term "core" often conjures images of sculpted abs and chiseled torsos. However, within the realm of Pilates, the concept of core goes far beyond mere aesthetics. It serves as the cornerstone of strength, stability, and alignment, providing a solid foundation upon which all movement is built.

Anatomy of the Core

Before we can fully grasp the significance of the core in Pilates, it's essential to understand its anatomical structure. At its core (pun intended), the core encompasses a complex network of muscles that extend beyond the superficial abdominals to include the deeper stabilizing muscles of the pelvis, hips, and spine. These muscles work in concert to provide support, stability, and mobility in every movement we undertake.

The Powerhouse: Centering in Pilates

In Pilates, the core is often referred to as the "powerhouse," a term coined by Joseph Pilates himself. This powerhouse serves as the focal point of all movement, acting as the center of gravity and source of strength for the entire body. By engaging the deep muscles of the core, practitioners cultivate stability and control, allowing for fluid and efficient movement with minimal strain on the joints.

Core Engagement in Pilates Exercises

Central to the Pilates method is the concept of initiating movement from the core. Whether performing a simple pelvic tilt or a complex series of exercises on the reformer, every movement begins with a deep connection to the powerhouse. Through precise alignment and controlled engagement of the core muscles, practitioners develop a heightened awareness of their body and its capabilities.

Benefits of Core Strength

The benefits of developing a strong and resilient core extend far beyond the confines of the Pilates studio. A stable core not only improves posture and alignment but also enhances functional movement patterns, reducing the risk of injury and improving athletic performance. Moreover, a strong core can alleviate back pain, improve balance, and enhance overall quality of life.

Cultivating Core Awareness

As we journey deeper into the world of Pilates, we will explore various exercises and techniques designed to awaken and strengthen the core. From foundational mat exercises to dynamic movements on the equipment, each exercise serves to deepen our understanding of the powerhouse and its role in fostering physical and mental wellbeing.

Join me as we embark on a journey to unlock the secrets of the core in Pilates, and discover the transformative power of strength, stability, and alignment from within.

Chapter 3: Mat Pilates: Essential Exercises for Strength and Flexibility

In the heart of the Pilates practice lies the foundation of Mat Pilates, a series of exercises designed to sculpt and strengthen the body using nothing more than a mat and the power of one's own body weight. Accessible to practitioners of all levels, Mat Pilates offers a pathway to improved strength, flexibility, and mind-body connection without the need for specialized equipment.

The Essence of Mat Pilates

Mat Pilates traces its roots back to the early days of Joseph Pilates' pioneering work, where he developed a series of floor exercises to help rehabilitate injured soldiers during World War I. Today, Mat Pilates remains a cornerstone of the Pilates method, offering a comprehensive workout that targets every muscle group while emphasizing proper alignment and control.

Principles of Mat Pilates

At the heart of Mat Pilates are the core principles that guide every movement and breath. From the focus on centering and precision to the principles of control and flow, each element serves to unite mind and body in a seamless integration of movement and breath. By adhering to these principles, practitioners can maximize the effectiveness of their workout and minimize the risk of injury.

Key Exercises in Mat Pilates

Mat Pilates features a diverse repertoire of exercises that target the entire body, from the powerhouse of the core to the extremities of the arms and legs. From classic exercises like the Hundred and the Roll-Up to more advanced movements such as the Teaser and the Swan, each exercise offers a unique challenge that promotes strength, flexibility, and coordination.

The Mind-Body Connection

One of the hallmarks of Mat Pilates is its emphasis on cultivating a deep connection between mind and body. Through mindful movement and breath awareness, practitioners learn to move with intention and precision, fostering a sense of presence and mindfulness that extends beyond the mat and into everyday life.

Creating Your Mat Pilates Practice

Whether you're a beginner looking to build strength and flexibility or an experienced practitioner seeking to deepen your practice, Mat Pilates offers a pathway to transformation for all. With its accessibility and versatility, Mat Pilates can be practiced virtually anywhere, making it an ideal addition to any fitness routine.

Join me as we explore the world of Mat Pilates, uncovering the secrets to a strong, flexible, and balanced body from the comfort of your own mat.

Chapter 4: Equipment-Based Pilates: Reformer, Cadillac, and More

While Mat Pilates forms the foundation of the practice, equipment-based Pilates adds a new dimension to the workout, offering endless possibilities for resistance, assistance, and refinement. From the iconic reformer to the versatile Cadillac and beyond, equipment-based Pilates provides a dynamic and transformative experience that challenges the body in new and exciting ways.

Evolution of Pilates Equipment

The evolution of Pilates equipment mirrors the evolution of the method itself, with each apparatus designed to enhance the effectiveness of the workout and target specific muscle groups. From Joseph Pilates' early inventions to the modern-day equipment found in Pilates studios around the world, each piece serves a unique purpose in sculpting and strengthening the body.

The Reformer: A Pilates Icon

At the heart of equipment-based Pilates lies the reformer, a versatile apparatus that provides resistance through a system of springs, pulleys, and straps. With its sliding carriage and adjustable springs, the reformer offers endless possibilities for resistance training, flexibility work, and core strengthening. From beginner-friendly exercises to advanced movements, the reformer provides a challenging yet supportive environment for practitioners of all levels.

The Cadillac: Versatility and Variability

Often referred to as the "Cadillac" due to its resemblance to a four-poster bed, this apparatus offers a wide range of exercises that target every muscle group in the body. From leg springs to push-through bars, the Cadillac provides endless opportunities for resistance training, stretching, and alignment work. With its elevated platform and adjustable springs, the Cadillac offers a dynamic and challenging workout that can be customized to suit individual needs and abilities.

Other Pilates Equipment

In addition to the reformer and Cadillac, there are a variety of other apparatus used in equipment-based Pilates, including the Wunda Chair, the Barrel, and the Spine Corrector. Each piece offers unique benefits and challenges, allowing practitioners to tailor their workout to target specific areas of the body or address individual needs.

Creating Your Equipment-Based Pilates Practice

Whether you're a seasoned Pilates enthusiast or new to the practice, equipment-based Pilates offers a transformative experience that challenges the body and invigorates the mind. With its endless possibilities for customization and progression, equipment-based Pilates provides a pathway to strength, flexibility, and alignment that goes beyond the confines of traditional exercise.

Join me as we explore the world of equipment-based Pilates, uncovering the secrets to a strong, supple, and balanced body through the power of resistance, assistance, and refinement.

Chapter 5: Breathing Techniques: Enhancing Mind-Body Connection

In the practice of Pilates, breath is the bridge that connects mind and body, uniting movement with intention and fostering a deep sense of presence and mindfulness. From the moment we step onto the mat or apparatus, the rhythm of our breath guides us through each movement, providing support, energy, and focus. In this chapter, we will explore the importance of breath in Pilates and learn how to harness its power to enhance our practice.

The Role of Breath in Pilates

Breath is not simply a physiological function; it is a fundamental aspect of the Pilates method. Joseph Pilates himself emphasized the importance of breath in facilitating movement, advocating for a deep, diaphragmatic breath that engages the entire torso and supports the core muscles. By synchronizing breath with movement, practitioners can enhance their control, stability, and precision, unlocking the full potential of each exercise.

The Three-Dimensional Breath

In Pilates, breath is often described as three-dimensional, encompassing not only the expansion and contraction of the rib cage but also the movement of the diaphragm and the engagement of the pelvic floor. By cultivating awareness of the breath in all three dimensions, practitioners can access a deeper level of connection to their core and enhance the effectiveness of their movements.

Breathing Techniques in Mat Pilates

In Mat Pilates, breath serves as a guide for movement, providing rhythm and flow to the exercises. From the initiation of movement on the inhale to the engagement of the core on the exhale, each breath is an integral part of the sequence, enhancing control, stability, and alignment. By paying attention to the quality and timing of their breath, practitioners can optimize their performance and maximize the benefits of their workout.

Breathing Techniques in Equipment-Based Pilates

In equipment-based Pilates, breath takes on added significance as practitioners navigate the resistance and assistance provided by the apparatus. Whether performing a movement on the reformer, Cadillac, or other equipment, breath serves as a constant companion, guiding and supporting the body through each exercise. By maintaining a steady and controlled breath, practitioners can harness the power of their breath to deepen their connection to their core and enhance their overall performance.

Mindful Breathing Beyond the Studio

As we delve deeper into the world of Pilates, we discover that the benefits of mindful breathing extend far beyond the confines of the studio. By cultivating a conscious awareness of our breath in everyday life, we can reduce stress, improve focus, and enhance our overall sense of wellbeing. Whether sitting at our desk, standing in line, or walking in nature, the breath serves as a constant reminder of our innate connection to the present moment.

Join me as we explore the transformative power of breath in Pilates, unlocking the secrets to greater control, stability, and presence both on and off the mat.

Chapter 6: Pilates for Rehabilitation and Injury Prevention

In the realm of fitness and wellness, Pilates stands out as a versatile and effective tool for rehabilitation and injury prevention. With its focus on alignment, stability, and controlled movement, Pilates offers a safe and gentle approach to restoring function, relieving pain, and preventing future injuries. In this chapter, we will explore the unique benefits of Pilates for rehabilitation and injury prevention and learn how it can be tailored to address specific conditions and concerns.

The Healing Power of Pilates
Pilates was originally developed by Joseph Pilates as a method of rehabilitation for injured soldiers during World War I. Today, it continues to be recognized as a valuable tool for addressing a wide range of musculoskeletal issues, from back pain and joint injuries to post-surgical recovery and chronic conditions. By emphasizing proper alignment, core stability, and controlled movement, Pilates provides a safe and effective environment for restoring function and promoting healing.

Adapting Pilates for Rehabilitation

One of the greatest strengths of Pilates lies in its adaptability and versatility. Whether recovering from surgery, managing a chronic condition, or recovering from an acute injury, Pilates can be tailored to meet the unique needs and abilities of each individual. By working closely with a qualified instructor or physical therapist, practitioners can develop a customized Pilates program that addresses their specific goals, concerns, and limitations.

Pilates for Common Injuries and Conditions

From low back pain and sciatica to shoulder impingement and knee injuries, Pilates offers targeted exercises and techniques to address a wide range of musculoskeletal issues. By focusing on strengthening weak muscles, improving flexibility, and correcting imbalances, Pilates can help alleviate pain, improve function, and prevent future injuries. Additionally, Pilates can be beneficial for conditions such as osteoporosis, arthritis, and fibromyalgia, providing gentle yet effective movement therapy for individuals with chronic pain and mobility issues.

Injury Prevention Through Pilates

Beyond its rehabilitative benefits, Pilates also plays a crucial role in injury prevention. By developing core strength, improving flexibility, and enhancing body awareness, Pilates helps individuals move with greater ease and efficiency, reducing the risk of overuse injuries and strain. Moreover, Pilates encourages mindful movement and proper alignment, empowering practitioners to move with awareness and intention in their daily activities, thus minimizing the risk of injury and promoting long-term musculoskeletal health.

Incorporating Pilates into Rehabilitation Programs

Whether as a standalone treatment or as part of a comprehensive rehabilitation program, Pilates can play a valuable role in promoting recovery and preventing future injuries. By integrating Pilates exercises and principles into physical therapy sessions, individuals can accelerate their healing process, improve their functional outcomes, and regain confidence in their bodies. Moreover, by continuing their Pilates practice beyond the rehabilitation phase, individuals can maintain their gains, prevent relapse, and enjoy lasting improvements in their overall health and wellbeing.

Join me as we explore the transformative potential of Pilates for rehabilitation and injury prevention, unlocking the secrets to healing, strength, and resilience from within.

Chapter 7: Pilates for Specific Populations: Pregnancy, Seniors, Athletes

Pilates is a versatile and adaptable practice that can be modified to suit the needs and abilities of diverse populations. From pregnant women seeking to maintain strength and flexibility to seniors looking to improve balance and mobility, and from athletes striving to enhance performance to individuals managing chronic conditions, Pilates offers a safe and effective way to achieve health and wellness goals. In this chapter, we will explore how Pilates can be tailored to address the unique needs of specific populations, empowering individuals of all ages and backgrounds to reap the benefits of this transformative practice.

Pilates During Pregnancy

Pregnancy is a time of profound physical and emotional changes, and Pilates can be a valuable tool for supporting women throughout this journey. By focusing on core stability, pelvic alignment, and breath awareness, Pilates helps pregnant women maintain strength, flexibility, and balance while reducing discomfort and preparing for childbirth. Modified exercises and mindful movement techniques ensure safety and comfort, allowing women to stay active and connected to their bodies throughout pregnancy and beyond.

Pilates for Seniors

As we age, maintaining strength, flexibility, and balance becomes increasingly important for overall health and wellbeing. Pilates offers a gentle yet effective approach to senior fitness, providing low-impact exercises that promote joint mobility, muscle strength, and postural alignment. By focusing on functional movement patterns and mindful breathing, Pilates helps seniors improve their quality of life, reduce the risk of falls, and maintain independence as they age.

Pilates for Athletes

Athletes of all levels can benefit from incorporating Pilates into their training regimen. By targeting specific muscle groups, improving flexibility, and enhancing body awareness, Pilates helps athletes improve performance, prevent injuries, and recover more quickly from intense training sessions. Whether training for a marathon, competing in a team sport, or pursuing individual fitness goals, athletes can use Pilates to enhance their strength, endurance, and agility, giving them a competitive edge on and off the field.

Pilates for Chronic Conditions

Pilates can also be a valuable resource for individuals managing chronic conditions such as back pain, arthritis, or fibromyalgia. By focusing on gentle, controlled movements and mindful breathing, Pilates helps alleviate pain, improve mobility, and enhance overall quality of life. Additionally, Pilates promotes relaxation and stress reduction, providing a holistic approach to managing chronic conditions and promoting overall health and wellbeing.

Tailoring Pilates for Specific Needs

Regardless of age, fitness level, or health status, Pilates can be customized to meet the unique needs and goals of each individual. Qualified instructors can adapt exercises, modify equipment, and provide personalized guidance to ensure a safe and effective workout for every client. Whether seeking rehabilitation, athletic enhancement, or simply a way to stay active and healthy, Pilates offers something for everyone, empowering individuals to achieve their full potential and live their best lives.

Join me as we explore the transformative potential of Pilates for specific populations, unlocking the secrets to health, vitality, and wellbeing for individuals of all ages and backgrounds.

Chapter 8: Integrating Pilates into Daily Life: Workouts and Routines

Pilates isn't just a workout; it's a way of life. With its focus on mindful movement, breath awareness, and body alignment, Pilates offers a holistic approach to health and wellbeing that extends far beyond the confines of the studio. In this chapter, we will explore practical strategies for integrating Pilates into daily life, from quick workouts that can be done at home or in the office to mindful movement practices that promote relaxation and stress relief throughout the day.

Morning Wake-Up Routine

Start your day off right with a Pilates-inspired morning routine designed to awaken the body, energize the mind, and set a positive tone for the day ahead. Incorporate gentle stretches, dynamic movements, and breath awareness exercises to increase circulation, improve flexibility, and enhance mental clarity. Whether it's a series of spinal rolls, a few rounds of the Hundred, or a simple breathing exercise, taking a few moments each morning to connect with your body can make a world of difference in how you feel throughout the day.

Midday Pick-Me-Up

Feeling sluggish or stressed in the middle of the day? Take a break from your desk or daily activities and indulge in a quick Pilates-inspired pick-me-up. Whether it's a brisk walk around the block, a few minutes of stretching at your desk, or a series of Pilates mat exercises in the break room, incorporating movement into your midday routine can help boost energy levels, improve focus, and relieve tension in the body and mind.

Evening Wind-Down Ritual

As the day draws to a close, take time to unwind and decompress with a gentle Pilates-inspired evening ritual. Incorporate restorative stretches, calming breathwork, and relaxation exercises to release tension, quiet the mind, and prepare for a restful night's sleep. Whether it's a series of gentle stretches on the mat, a relaxing foam rolling session, or a few minutes of meditation before bed, prioritizing self-care and relaxation can help promote deep rest and rejuvenation for body and soul.

Incorporating Pilates into Daily Activities

In addition to dedicated workouts and routines, look for opportunities to integrate Pilates principles into your daily activities. Whether it's sitting at your desk, standing in line, or walking down the street, practice mindful posture, deep breathing, and core engagement to promote alignment, stability, and body awareness throughout the day. By bringing the principles of Pilates into every aspect of your life, you can cultivate a deeper connection to your body, enhance your physical health, and promote overall wellbeing.

Making Pilates a Priority

Ultimately, integrating Pilates into daily life is about making it a priority and finding creative ways to incorporate movement, mindfulness, and self-care into your routine. Whether it's a quick workout in the morning, a midday stretch break, or a mindful movement practice before bed, carving out time for Pilates amidst the busyness of life can have profound benefits for body, mind, and spirit. Remember, Pilates isn't just something you do; it's a way of being—a commitment to nurturing and honoring yourself each and every day.

Join me as we explore the art of integrating Pilates into daily life, unlocking the secrets to health, vitality, and wellbeing for body and soul.

Chapter 9: The Science Behind Pilates: How It Benefits the Body

Pilates isn't just a fitness trend—it's a scientifically backed method for enhancing physical and mental wellbeing. From improving strength and flexibility to promoting relaxation and stress reduction, Pilates offers a wealth of benefits that are supported by research and scientific evidence. In this chapter, we will explore the science behind Pilates and uncover the physiological and psychological mechanisms that underlie its transformative effects on the body and mind.

Muscle Activation and Strength

At the core of Pilates is a focus on strengthening the deep stabilizing muscles of the core, including the transverse abdominis, pelvic floor, and multifidus. Research has shown that Pilates exercises effectively activate these muscles, leading to improvements in core strength, stability, and postural alignment. Additionally, Pilates targets major muscle groups throughout the body, including the abdominals, back, hips, and shoulders, resulting in balanced muscular development and enhanced functional movement patterns.

Flexibility and Range of Motion

Pilates incorporates dynamic stretching and controlled movement patterns that promote flexibility and joint mobility. Research has demonstrated that regular Pilates practice can lead to improvements in flexibility, particularly in key areas such as the hamstrings, hips, and spine. By lengthening and elongating the muscles through a combination of stretching and strengthening exercises, Pilates helps improve range of motion and reduce the risk of injury.

Posture and Alignment

Poor posture is a common problem in today's sedentary society, leading to a host of musculoskeletal issues such as back pain, neck tension, and joint dysfunction. Pilates emphasizes proper alignment and postural awareness, teaching practitioners to engage the core, stabilize the spine, and maintain neutral alignment throughout movement. Research has shown that Pilates can lead to improvements in posture, resulting in reduced pain and discomfort and improved overall quality of life.

Balance and Stability

Balance and stability are essential components of functional movement and injury prevention. Pilates exercises challenge proprioception and balance, requiring practitioners to engage the core and stabilize the body in various positions and movements. Research has shown that Pilates can improve balance and stability, particularly in older adults and individuals with neurological conditions such as Parkinson's disease. By enhancing proprioception and body awareness, Pilates helps reduce the risk of falls and improve confidence in movement.

Mindfulness and Stress Reduction

Beyond its physical benefits, Pilates offers a pathway to mental wellbeing through mindfulness and stress reduction. The focus on breath awareness, body connection, and present-moment awareness cultivates a state of mindfulness that promotes relaxation and stress relief. Research has shown that Pilates can reduce levels of stress hormones such as cortisol, leading to improvements in mood, sleep quality, and overall psychological wellbeing.

The Holistic Approach of Pilates

What sets Pilates apart from other forms of exercise is its holistic approach to health and wellness. By addressing the interconnectedness of mind, body, and spirit, Pilates offers a comprehensive framework for achieving optimal health and vitality. From its emphasis on core strength and flexibility to its promotion of mindfulness and stress reduction, Pilates provides a multifaceted approach to fitness that supports the whole person—physically, mentally, and emotionally.

Join me as we explore the science behind Pilates, uncovering the physiological and psychological mechanisms that make it such a powerful tool for enhancing health, vitality, and wellbeing.

Chapter 10: Mindfulness and Pilates: Cultivating Mental Wellbeing

In a world filled with distractions and demands, finding moments of peace and presence can seem like a rare luxury. Yet, within the practice of Pilates lies a pathway to mindfulness—a state of being that brings attention to the present moment with acceptance and non-judgment. In this chapter, we will explore how Pilates serves as a vehicle for cultivating mindfulness, fostering a deep connection between mind and body that enhances mental wellbeing and enriches the overall Pilates experience.

The Mind-Body Connection in Pilates

At its core, Pilates is about more than just physical fitness; it's about forging a deep and intimate connection between mind and body. Through mindful movement, breath awareness, and focused attention, Pilates practitioners learn to inhabit their bodies fully, tuning in to the sensations, thoughts, and emotions that arise with each movement. By cultivating this mind-body connection, Pilates becomes not just a workout, but a journey of self-discovery and self-awareness.

Breath as the Bridge to Mindfulness

One of the primary tools for cultivating mindfulness in Pilates is the breath. Joseph Pilates himself emphasized the importance of breath as a guiding force for movement, advocating for a deep, diaphragmatic breath that engages the entire torso. By syncing breath with movement, practitioners learn to harness the power of the breath to quiet the mind, release tension, and cultivate a sense of calm and presence. Whether performing a simple exercise on the mat or navigating a challenging sequence on the reformer, the breath serves as a constant anchor, grounding practitioners in the present moment and fostering a deep sense of mindfulness.

Body Awareness and Sensory Perception

In Pilates, every movement is an opportunity to deepen our awareness of the body and its sensations. By paying close attention to the alignment, engagement, and execution of each exercise, practitioners develop a heightened sense of body awareness that extends beyond the mat and into everyday life. Through mindful movement and sensory perception, Pilates becomes a practice of self-inquiry and self-discovery, allowing practitioners to uncover hidden tensions, release limiting beliefs, and cultivate a greater sense of freedom and ease in their bodies.

Presence and Acceptance

Central to the practice of mindfulness is the cultivation of presence and acceptance—the ability to be fully present with whatever arises in the moment, without judgment or resistance. In Pilates, this means embracing the body exactly as it is, with all its imperfections, limitations, and strengths. By approaching each movement with curiosity, openness, and acceptance, practitioners learn to let go of striving and perfectionism, and instead cultivate a sense of ease, grace, and joy in their practice.

The Transformative Power of Mindfulness in Pilates

As we journey deeper into the practice of Pilates, we discover that the true magic lies not in the physical exercises themselves, but in the mindful awareness with which we approach them. By cultivating mindfulness on the mat, we develop the capacity to navigate life's challenges with greater ease, resilience, and grace. Whether it's finding stillness in a moment of chaos, or finding strength in a moment of weakness, Pilates becomes a sanctuary—a refuge where mind, body, and spirit converge in perfect harmony.

Join me as we explore the transformative power of mindfulness in Pilates, unlocking the secrets to greater presence, peace, and wellbeing both on and off the mat.

Chapter 11: Advanced Pilates: Challenging Exercises and Progressions

For those who have mastered the fundamentals of Pilates and are hungry for a greater challenge, advanced Pilates offers a rich tapestry of exercises and techniques to push the boundaries of strength, flexibility, and control. From dynamic movements that test endurance and coordination to advanced exercises on the reformer, Cadillac, and other equipment, advanced Pilates provides a pathway to deeper exploration and transformation. In this chapter, we will delve into the world of advanced Pilates, exploring the key principles, exercises, and progressions that define this dynamic and exhilarating practice.

Mastering the Principles

At the heart of advanced Pilates lies a deep understanding of the core principles that govern the method. From centering and precision to control and flow, each principle serves as a guiding light, illuminating the path to mastery and refinement. By honing these principles with precision and intention, practitioners lay the foundation for advanced Pilates, unlocking the secrets to greater strength, flexibility, and control.

Dynamic Movement Sequences

Advanced Pilates is characterized by dynamic movement sequences that challenge the body in new and exciting ways. From flowing transitions between exercises to complex combinations that target multiple muscle groups simultaneously, advanced Pilates requires practitioners to move with grace, fluidity, and precision. By mastering the art of sequencing, practitioners learn to create seamless transitions between exercises, maximizing the efficiency and effectiveness of their workouts.

Advanced Mat Exercises

While Mat Pilates forms the foundation of the practice, advanced practitioners can take their mat work to new heights with a variety of challenging exercises and progressions. From advanced variations of classic exercises like the Roll-Up and the Teaser to dynamic movements such as the Control Balance and the Boomerang, advanced mat work offers a full-body workout that tests strength, flexibility, and control.

Advanced Equipment-Based Exercises

In addition to mat work, advanced Pilates practitioners can explore a wide range of advanced exercises on the reformer, Cadillac, and other equipment. From advanced variations of familiar exercises to specialized movements that target specific muscle groups, advanced equipment-based Pilates offers endless possibilities for challenging and transformative workouts. Whether it's performing a series of advanced footwork exercises on the reformer or

executing a complex sequence on the Cadillac, advanced
practitioners can push the boundaries of their practice and
achieve new levels of strength, flexibility, and control.

Progressions and Modifications

As with any advanced practice, it's important for
practitioners to progress gradually and mindfully, listening
to their bodies and honoring their limitations. Advanced
Pilates exercises can be challenging and demanding,
requiring a solid foundation of strength, flexibility, and
body awareness. By working with a qualified instructor and
gradually introducing advanced exercises and progressions
into their practice, practitioners can safely and effectively
expand their repertoire and achieve their fitness goals.

The Journey of Mastery

Advanced Pilates is not just about mastering challenging
exercises—it's about embarking on a journey of self-
discovery and personal growth. As practitioners delve
deeper into the practice, they discover new layers of
strength, flexibility, and control within themselves,
unlocking the true potential of their bodies and minds.
Whether it's conquering a challenging exercise for the first
time or experiencing a breakthrough in body awareness,
advanced Pilates offers endless opportunities for growth,
exploration, and transformation.

Join me as we explore the exhilarating world of advanced Pilates, unlocking the secrets to mastery, refinement, and transformation for body, mind, and spirit.

Chapter 12: Beyond the Studio: Applying Pilates Principles in Everyday Life

While the studio serves as the primary space for Pilates practice, the principles and benefits of Pilates can extend far beyond the confines of the mat or apparatus. In this chapter, we will explore how Pilates principles can be applied in everyday life, empowering practitioners to cultivate strength, flexibility, and mindfulness in all aspects of their lives.

Posture and Alignment

One of the most tangible benefits of Pilates is improved posture and alignment. By focusing on core strength, spinal alignment, and body awareness in the studio, practitioners develop habits that carry over into everyday life. Whether sitting at a desk, standing in line, or walking down the street, Pilates practitioners can apply the principles of alignment to maintain a tall, upright posture and reduce strain on the spine and joints.

Functional Movement

Pilates emphasizes functional movement patterns that mimic activities of daily living, such as bending, twisting, reaching, and lifting. By practicing these movements in the studio, practitioners develop strength, flexibility, and coordination that translate into improved performance in everyday activities. Whether picking up groceries, playing with children, or gardening in the yard, Pilates practitioners can move with greater ease, efficiency, and confidence in their daily lives.

Breath Awareness

The breath is a central focus of Pilates, serving as a bridge between mind and body and a source of energy and vitality. By cultivating breath awareness in the studio, practitioners learn to harness the power of the breath to reduce stress, increase focus, and promote relaxation. Whether facing a challenging situation at work, navigating a difficult conversation, or simply dealing with the ups and downs of daily life, Pilates practitioners can use breath awareness to stay centered, grounded, and present in the moment.

Mindful Movement

Pilates encourages mindful movement—a state of focused attention and awareness that brings greater depth and meaning to each moment. By practicing mindful movement in the studio, practitioners learn to approach life with a sense of curiosity, openness, and acceptance. Whether eating a meal, taking a walk, or spending time with loved ones, Pilates practitioners can bring the same level of presence and intention to their daily activities, enhancing their overall sense of wellbeing and fulfillment.

Self-Care and Wellbeing

Above all, Pilates teaches the importance of self-care and wellbeing—a commitment to nurturing and honoring oneself on a physical, mental, and emotional level. By prioritizing self-care practices such as regular exercise, healthy nutrition, adequate rest, and stress management, Pilates practitioners create a foundation for health and happiness that extends far beyond the studio. Whether practicing Pilates or engaging in other self-care activities, practitioners can cultivate a greater sense of balance, resilience, and vitality in all aspects of their lives.

Community and Connection

Finally, Pilates fosters a sense of community and connection that extends beyond the studio walls. Whether participating in group classes, attending workshops, or connecting with fellow practitioners online, Pilates offers opportunities for friendship, support, and camaraderie that enrich the overall Pilates experience. By building relationships with like-minded individuals who share a passion for health and wellness, Pilates practitioners create a sense of belonging and connection that enhances their journey of self-discovery and personal growth.

Join me as we explore the transformative potential of Pilates beyond the studio, unlocking the secrets to health, happiness, and fulfillment in everyday life.

Chapter 13: FAQs and Common Misconceptions About Pilates

As Pilates continues to gain popularity around the world, it's natural for people to have questions and misconceptions about this dynamic and transformative practice. In this chapter, we'll address some of the most common inquiries and clear up any misconceptions to help you better understand the principles, benefits, and applications of Pilates.

1. What is Pilates?

Pilates is a mind-body exercise system developed by Joseph Pilates in the early 20th century. It focuses on strengthening the core muscles, improving flexibility, and enhancing body awareness through controlled movements and breath awareness.

2. Is Pilates only for women?

No, Pilates is for everyone! While it's true that Pilates was originally developed by a man, Joseph Pilates, and gained popularity among dancers, it is suitable for people of all ages, genders, and fitness levels.

3. Do I need to be flexible to do Pilates?

No, flexibility is not a prerequisite for Pilates. Pilates can actually help improve flexibility over time through gentle stretching and controlled movement. Practitioners can start at their own level and gradually progress as their flexibility increases.

4. Will Pilates help me lose weight?

While Pilates can contribute to weight loss when combined with a healthy diet and regular cardiovascular exercise, its primary focus is on building strength, improving flexibility, and enhancing overall fitness. Many people find that Pilates helps tone and sculpt their bodies, leading to a more streamlined appearance.

5. Can I do Pilates if I have back pain?

Yes, Pilates can be beneficial for people with back pain, as it focuses on strengthening the core muscles that support the spine and improving overall posture. However, it's important to work with a qualified instructor who can tailor the exercises to your individual needs and ensure proper alignment and technique.

6. Do I need special equipment to do Pilates?

While Pilates can be practiced using specialized equipment such as reformers, Cadillacs, and chairs, it can also be done using just a mat. Mat Pilates exercises use body weight as resistance and can be performed virtually anywhere, making it accessible to everyone.

7. How often should I do Pilates?

The frequency of Pilates practice depends on individual goals, preferences, and schedules. Some people benefit from practicing Pilates several times a week, while others may find that one or two sessions per week is sufficient to see results. Consistency is key, so it's important to find a routine that works for you and stick with it.

8. Can I do Pilates if I'm pregnant?

Yes, Pilates can be safe and beneficial during pregnancy when practiced under the guidance of a qualified instructor who specializes in prenatal Pilates. Modified exercises and careful attention to body alignment can help pregnant women maintain strength, flexibility, and comfort throughout their pregnancy.

9. Will Pilates make me bulky?

No, Pilates is not designed to build bulky muscles. Instead, it focuses on creating long, lean muscles through controlled movements and proper alignment. Many people find that Pilates helps improve muscle tone and definition without adding bulk.

10. Is Pilates similar to yoga?

While Pilates and yoga share some similarities, such as a focus on breath awareness and mind-body connection, they are distinct practices with different principles and objectives. Pilates emphasizes core strength, functional movement, and precise alignment, whereas yoga focuses more on flexibility, balance, and spiritual development.

By addressing these frequently asked questions and debunking common misconceptions, we hope to provide a clearer understanding of the principles, benefits, and applications of Pilates, empowering you to embark on your own Pilates journey with confidence and clarity.

Conclusion: Embracing the Pilates Journey

As we reach the end of our exploration into the world of
Pilates, it's clear that this practice is much more than just a
series of exercises—it's a journey of self-discovery,
transformation, and empowerment. From its humble
beginnings in a small New York City studio to its
widespread popularity around the globe, Pilates has
remained true to its core principles of strength, flexibility,
and mindfulness, offering a pathway to health, vitality, and
wellbeing for people of all ages and backgrounds.

Throughout this book, we've delved into the fundamental
principles of Pilates, explored its many benefits for the
body and mind, and examined its applications in various
contexts, from rehabilitation and injury prevention to
pregnancy and beyond. We've discovered how Pilates can
be adapted to suit the needs of specific populations,
integrated into daily life, and advanced to challenge even
the most seasoned practitioners.

But perhaps most importantly, we've come to understand
that Pilates is not just a workout—it's a way of life. It's
about cultivating strength, flexibility, and mindfulness in
all aspects of our lives, from the way we move and breathe
to the way we think and feel. It's about embracing our
bodies exactly as they are, with all their imperfections,
limitations, and strengths, and learning to move with grace,
ease, and intention.

As you embark on your own Pilates journey, remember that it's not about perfection—it's about progress. It's about showing up on the mat, day after day, with an open heart and a curious mind, ready to explore what your body is capable of and how it can serve you best. Whether you're a beginner just starting out or an advanced practitioner pushing the boundaries of your practice, know that Pilates has something to offer you, wherever you are on your journey.

So embrace the challenge, embrace the journey, and above all, embrace yourself. Because in the end, Pilates is not just about building a stronger body—it's about building a stronger, more resilient, and more empowered you.

Thank you for joining me on this journey into the world of Pilates. May your practice be filled with joy, discovery, and endless possibilities.